The Biohacking Guide

Mastering the Art of Optimizing Your Body and Mind

Bryan Sherrell

Bryan Sherrell

The Biohacking Guide: Mastering the Art of Optimizing Your Body and Mind

Cover design by Ali Genshaw

Printed in United States of America

Disclaimer

The information provided in this book is for educational and informational purposes only. While every effort has been made to ensure the accuracy and completeness of the content, the author/publisher makes no representations or warranties of any kind, express or implied, about the completeness, accuracy, reliability, suitability, or availability of the information contained herein.

The techniques, strategies, and suggestions presented in this book are based on the author's personal experiences and research. They may not be suitable for every individual or situation. Readers are advised to use their own discretion and judgment when applying any information from this book to their own circumstances.

The author/publisher shall not be held liable for any loss, injury, or damage arising from the use of the information contained in this book. Readers are solely responsible for their own actions and decisions.

Any references to specific products, services, or organizations are provided for informational purposes only and do not constitute an endorsement or recommendation. The author/publisher shall not be held liable for any consequences resulting from the use or misuse of such products, services, or organizations.

It is recommended that readers consult with qualified professionals or experts in the relevant field before making any significant decisions or taking any actions based on the information provided in this book.

By reading this book, the reader acknowledges and agrees to the terms of this disclaimer.

Dedication

To those who seek to unlock the full potential of their bodies and minds, this book is for you. May your journey towards health, happiness, and longevity be filled with curiosity, resilience, and boundless vitality. Here's to living your best life, for as long as possible.

Table of Content

Introduction: Unlocking Your Full Potential

- **The Biohacking Revolution**

- **Why Biohacking Matters**

- **How to Use This Guide**

- **The Biohacker's Mindset**

In the ever-evolving landscape of health and wellness, a new movement has emerged that challenges traditional approaches and empowers individuals to take control of their own biology. This movement is known as biohacking. Rooted in a desire to optimize the body and mind, biohacking is a practice that merges cutting-edge science, technology, and self-experimentation to push the boundaries of human potential. Whether you're seeking to enhance your cognitive abilities, improve your physical health, or extend your lifespan, biohacking offers a personalized, data-driven path to achieving your goals.

The origins of biohacking can be traced back to a convergence of several key influences: the rise of the quantified self-movement, advancements in technology, and a growing interest in alternative health practices. The quantified self-movement, which began in the early 2000s, encouraged people to track various aspects of their lives—such as sleep patterns, exercise routines, and dietary habits—using digital tools and wearable devices. This focus on self-tracking laid the groundwork for a more scientific approach to personal health, one that values data collection and analysis as a means of understanding and improving individual well-being.

At the same time, technological advancements have made it easier than ever to access information, conduct experiments, and monitor progress. From DNA testing kits that reveal genetic predispositions to smart devices that track biometrics in real-time, the tools available to modern biohackers are powerful and increasingly accessible. These technologies have democratized the field of personal health optimization, allowing anyone with the curiosity and determination to become their own health expert.

Biohacking also draws inspiration from alternative health practices, such as ancient meditation techniques, herbal medicine, and holistic approaches to wellness. By integrating these time-tested methods with modern science, biohackers aim to create a comprehensive approach to health that addresses both the physical and mental aspects of well-being. This blend of tradition and innovation is a hallmark of the biohacking philosophy, which seeks to combine the best of both worlds to achieve optimal results.

As the biohacking movement has grown, it has attracted a diverse community of enthusiasts, ranging from Silicon Valley entrepreneurs to professional athletes to everyday people who are simply passionate about improving their lives. What unites this community is a shared belief that we can and should take control of our own health destinies. Biohackers reject the notion that we are passive recipients of our genetic fate or that we must rely solely on conventional medicine to manage our health. Instead, they advocate for a proactive approach that involves experimenting with different strategies, tracking outcomes, and making informed decisions based on real data.

But why does biohacking matter? The answer lies in its potential to profoundly impact health, performance, and longevity. At its core, biohacking is about optimization—finding the most effective ways to enhance our bodies and minds so that we can live better, longer, and more fulfilling lives.

When it comes to health, biohacking offers tools and techniques for addressing a wide range of concerns, from boosting energy levels to managing chronic conditions to improving mental clarity. By understanding and manipulating the factors that influence our biology, biohackers can fine-tune their health in ways that were previously unimaginable. For example, a biohacker might use intermittent fasting to improve metabolic health, or they might incorporate nootropics—substances that enhance cognitive function—into their daily routine to sharpen focus and memory. These practices go beyond traditional health advice, offering personalized solutions that are tailored to an individual's unique biology and goals.

Performance is another key area where biohacking can make a significant difference. Whether you're an athlete looking to shave seconds off your personal best, a professional aiming to enhance productivity, or a student seeking to improve concentration, biohacking provides strategies for unlocking peak performance. Techniques such as optimizing sleep, adjusting nutrition, and employing mental training exercises can all contribute to better physical and cognitive performance. By systematically experimenting with these variables, biohackers can discover what works best for them and apply those insights to achieve their desired outcomes.

Perhaps the most compelling reason why biohacking matters is its potential to extend longevity and enhance the quality of life as we age. The quest for longevity has been a human pursuit for centuries, and biohacking represents the latest chapter in this ongoing story. By leveraging the latest research in genetics, nutrition, and regenerative medicine, biohackers are exploring ways to slow down the aging process, prevent age-related diseases, and even reverse some of the effects of aging. This is not about seeking immortality, but rather about maximizing the number of healthy, active years we have. In this sense, biohacking is not just about living longer; it's about living better for longer.

As you begin your journey into biohacking, it's important to understand how to navigate the wealth of information and techniques available to you. This guide is designed to be your companion on this journey, offering practical advice, evidence-based strategies, and insights from my knowledge in the field. Each chapter of this book delves into a specific aspect of biohacking, from sleep optimization to cognitive enhancement to environmental design. Along the way, you'll find tips for safely experimenting with different techniques, as well as suggestions for tracking and analyzing your progress.

To get the most out of this guide, approach it with an open

mind and a willingness to experiment. Biohacking is not a one-size-fits-all endeavor; what works for one person may not work for another. The key is to approach each technique with curiosity and a spirit of exploration. Start with small, manageable experiments, and pay close attention to how your body and mind respond. Use the tracking tools and methods described in this book to collect data on your progress, and don't be afraid to adjust your approach based on what you learn.

It's also important to remember that biohacking is an ongoing process, not a destination. The science of health and wellness is constantly evolving, and new discoveries are being made every day. As you continue on your biohacking journey, stay informed about the latest research and be open to adapting your strategies as new information becomes available. This guide is a starting point, but the true power of biohacking lies in your ability to continuously learn, experiment, and refine your approach over time.

At the heart of successful biohacking is a mindset that embraces curiosity, critical thinking, and adaptability. The biohacker's mindset is one of constant inquiry—an eagerness to ask questions, seek out new information, and challenge the status quo. Biohackers are not content to accept things at face value; they dig deeper, analyze data, and seek out evidence to support their decisions. This critical thinking is what sets biohacking apart from other health movements. It's not about following trends or adopting practices without understanding why they work; it's about making informed choices based on real science and personal experience.

Adaptability is another key component of the biohacker's mindset. The human body is incredibly complex, and what works today might not work tomorrow. Biohackers must be flexible, willing to adjust their strategies as new information emerges or as their bodies change. This adaptability is what allows biohackers to stay ahead of the curve and continue making progress toward their goals, even in the face of challenges or setbacks.

As you embark on your biohacking journey, keep these principles in mind. Embrace the spirit of experimentation, approach each technique with curiosity and critical thinking, and remain adaptable in the face of new information or changing circumstances. By adopting this mindset, you'll be well-equipped to unlock your full potential and achieve the health, performance, and longevity you desire.

In the chapters that follow, you'll find a wealth of information and practical advice to help you on your journey. From optimizing your sleep and nutrition to enhancing your cognitive function and physical fitness, this guide covers all the essential aspects of biohacking. Each chapter is designed to provide you with actionable strategies that you can start implementing right away. Whether you're new to biohacking or a seasoned practitioner, this guide offers valuable insights that will help you take your practice to the next level.

Welcome to the world of biohacking. The journey to unlocking your full potential begins here.

Chapter 1: The Foundations of Biohacking

- **Understanding the Basics**

- **Ethics and Safety**

- **Setting Personal Goals**

- **Tools of the Trade**

Biohacking, at its core, is the art and science of optimizing your body and mind through deliberate and strategic interventions. It's about taking control of your own biology, using a blend of science, technology, and a deep understanding of your body to achieve your desired outcomes. Whether your goal is to improve cognitive function, enhance physical performance, or extend your lifespan, biohacking provides a personalized roadmap to get you there. But before diving into specific techniques and strategies, it's crucial to understand the foundational concepts that underpin this practice.

At its most basic level, biohacking can be defined as the process of using science and technology to make measurable improvements in your body's performance, health, and overall well-being. The term itself may conjure images of futuristic technology or extreme self-experimentation, but the reality is that biohacking encompasses a wide range of practices, from the simple to the sophisticated. For some, biohacking might mean optimizing their diet and exercise routine, while for others, it might involve using wearable devices to track biometrics or even experimenting with advanced supplements and nootropics.

One of the key concepts in biohacking is self-experimentation. Unlike traditional approaches to health and wellness, which often rely on standardized guidelines and one-size-fits-all solutions, biohacking is highly individualized. It's about discovering what works best for you through trial and error. This means being willing to experiment with different techniques, track the results, and adjust your approach based on the data you collect. Self-experimentation requires a mindset of curiosity and openness, as well as a willingness to challenge assumptions and explore new possibilities.

Optimization is another central tenet of biohacking. The goal is not just to maintain health but to actively enhance and optimize it. This might involve fine-tuning your sleep patterns to improve cognitive function, adjusting your diet to boost energy levels, or developing a meditation practice to reduce stress and increase focus. The possibilities are endless, and the pursuit of optimization is what drives biohackers to continually push the boundaries of what's possible.

However, as with any practice that involves manipulating your body's systems, biohacking comes with its own set of ethical considerations and safety concerns. It's important to approach biohacking with a responsible and informed mindset, recognizing the potential risks as well as the benefits. One of the primary ethical considerations in biohacking is the concept of informed consent. When you engage in biohacking, you're essentially conducting experiments on yourself. This means that you need to be fully aware of the potential outcomes, both positive and negative, and make decisions that align with your personal values and risk tolerance.

Safety is another critical aspect of biohacking. While some biohacking practices are relatively low-risk, others can have significant implications for your health. For example, experimenting with new supplements or nootropics without fully understanding their effects can lead to unintended consequences. That's why it's essential to do your research, consult with professionals when necessary, and start with small, incremental changes rather than diving headfirst into more extreme interventions. Monitoring your body's response to these changes is crucial, as it allows you to make adjustments and avoid potential harm.

Setting personal goals is a key step in any biohacking journey. Biohacking is not a random collection of experiments but a targeted approach to achieving specific outcomes. To be successful, you need to have a clear understanding of what you want to accomplish. Are you looking to improve your mental clarity, increase your physical stamina, or enhance your overall well-being? Whatever your goals may be, it's important to define them clearly and make them measurable. This will not only give you direction but also allow you to track your progress and adjust your strategies as needed.

When setting goals, it's important to be realistic and specific. Rather than aiming for vague outcomes like "better health," focus on concrete objectives such as "improving sleep quality by tracking and adjusting bedtime routines" or "enhancing cognitive function by incorporating nootropics into my daily routine." Once you've defined your goals, break them down into smaller, manageable steps. This will make the process less overwhelming and increase your chances of success.

As you begin your biohacking journey, it's also helpful to establish a baseline for where you're starting from. This might involve tracking your current health metrics, such as weight, body fat percentage, or blood pressure, as well as assessing your cognitive function, energy levels, and overall sense of well-being. By establishing a baseline, you'll be able to measure the impact of your biohacking efforts and make data-driven decisions about what's working and what's not.

The tools and resources available to biohackers today are vast and varied, ranging from simple tracking apps to sophisticated wearable devices and genetic testing kits. These tools play a crucial role in helping you monitor your progress, collect data, and refine your approach. One of the most common tools in biohacking is the wearable device. Devices like fitness trackers, smartwatches, and heart rate monitors allow you to track a wide range of biometrics, including sleep patterns, heart rate variability, and physical activity levels. By analyzing this data, you can gain valuable insights into how your body responds to different interventions and make adjustments accordingly.

In addition to wearables, there are numerous apps designed to support your biohacking efforts. These apps can help you track your diet, monitor your exercise routines, manage stress, and even guide you through meditation practices. Some apps are specifically designed for biohackers, offering advanced features like biometric tracking, personalized recommendations, and integration with other health-related tools. The key is to choose the tools that align with your goals and provide the data and support you need to succeed.

For those looking to delve deeper into biohacking, there are also more advanced tools and resources available, such as genetic testing kits and lab testing services. Genetic testing can provide insights into your unique genetic makeup, helping you understand your predispositions to certain health conditions and guiding your biohacking efforts accordingly. Lab testing services allow you to monitor biomarkers like hormone levels, nutrient deficiencies, and inflammation markers, giving you a more comprehensive understanding of your health and enabling you to make targeted interventions.

As you explore the world of biohacking, it's important to remember that these tools are just that—tools. They are there to support and enhance your efforts, but they are not a substitute for common sense, critical thinking, and a well-rounded approach to health and wellness. Use them wisely, and always keep in mind the bigger picture of what you're trying to achieve.

In conclusion, the foundations of biohacking are built on

the principles of self-experimentation, optimization, ethics, safety, and goal setting. By understanding and applying these principles, you can embark on a biohacking journey that is both effective and sustainable. The tools and resources available today make it easier than ever to track your progress, gather data, and refine your approach. However, the true power of biohacking lies in your ability to take control of your own health and make informed decisions that align with your personal goals and values.

As you move forward, remember that biohacking is not about perfection or achieving instant results. It's about continuous learning, experimentation, and growth. The more you engage with the process, the more you'll discover about yourself and what you're capable of achieving. So, take that first step, set your goals, and embrace the journey of optimizing your body and mind. The possibilities are endless, and the rewards are well worth the effort.

Chapter 2: Optimizing Sleep for Peak Performance

- **The Science of Sleep**

- **Sleep Hacks for Better Rest**

- **Advanced Sleep Techniques**

- **Tracking and Analyzing Sleep**

Sleep is often underestimated, but it is one of the most critical factors in achieving peak performance, both mentally and physically. The quality of your sleep directly influences your ability to learn, remember, and execute tasks, as well as your overall health and well-being. To truly unlock your full potential, mastering the art of sleep optimization is essential. This chapter delves into the science of sleep, practical strategies for improving sleep quality, advanced techniques for those looking to push the boundaries of conventional sleep, and the importance of tracking and analyzing your sleep data to continually refine your approach.

The Science of Sleep

To fully appreciate the importance of sleep, it's crucial to understand the basic science behind it. Sleep is not a uniform state of rest but a complex, dynamic process that involves several stages, each playing a distinct role in your overall health and recovery.

Sleep is divided into two main types: Rapid Eye Movement (REM) sleep and Non-REM (NREM) sleep. NREM sleep is further broken down into three stages, each progressively deeper than the last. The first stage of NREM sleep is a light sleep, where you can be easily awakened. This stage is a transition from wakefulness to sleep and typically lasts only a few minutes. The second stage is a deeper form of light sleep, where your body temperature drops, your heart rate slows, and your body begins the process of physical recovery. This stage is important for consolidating memories and is where you spend the majority of your sleep time.

The third stage of NREM sleep, also known as deep sleep or slow-wave sleep, is the most restorative. During this stage, your body repairs tissues, builds bone and muscle, and strengthens the immune system. Deep sleep is crucial for physical recovery and overall health, and it's the stage that leaves you feeling refreshed and energized in the morning.

REM sleep, on the other hand, is the stage where dreaming occurs. During REM sleep, your brain is highly active, almost as much as when you're awake. This stage is critical for cognitive functions such as memory consolidation, learning, and emotional processing. REM sleep also plays a role in creativity and problem-solving. The cycles of REM and NREM sleep alternate throughout the night, with REM periods becoming longer as the night progresses. A full sleep cycle typically lasts about 90 minutes, and it's normal to experience four to six cycles per night.

Understanding these stages is important because each one contributes uniquely to your overall well-being. Disruptions in any stage can affect your performance the next day. For example, a lack of deep sleep can leave you feeling physically tired, while insufficient REM sleep can impair cognitive function and emotional resilience. Therefore, optimizing your sleep means ensuring that you not only get enough sleep but also achieve a balanced distribution across these stages.

Sleep Hacks for Better Rest

Optimizing your sleep starts with establishing good sleep hygiene and creating an environment conducive to rest.

Sleep hygiene refers to the habits and practices that are necessary for getting quality sleep on a regular basis. The foundation of good sleep hygiene includes maintaining a consistent sleep schedule, creating a relaxing bedtime routine, and ensuring that your sleep environment is comfortable and free from distractions.

One of the most effective sleep hacks is to maintain a regular sleep schedule. Going to bed and waking up at the same time every day, even on weekends, helps regulate your body's internal clock, making it easier to fall asleep and wake up naturally. This consistency reinforces your circadian rhythm, the 24-hour cycle that influences many physiological processes, including sleep.

Another crucial aspect of sleep hygiene is managing your exposure to light, especially in the evening. Light, particularly blue light emitted by screens on phones, tablets, and computers, can interfere with the production of melatonin, the hormone that signals your body that it's time to sleep. To improve sleep quality, it's recommended to reduce screen time at least an hour before bed. Instead, opt for activities that help you wind down, such as reading a book, taking a warm bath, or practicing relaxation techniques like meditation or deep breathing exercises.

Your sleep environment also plays a significant role in determining the quality of your rest. Your bedroom should be cool, quiet, and dark to create the ideal conditions for sleep. Investing in a comfortable mattress and pillows can make a big difference in how well you sleep. Additionally, consider using blackout curtains or a sleep mask to block out light, and earplugs or a white noise machine to mask any disruptive sounds.

Temperature regulation is another key factor. The body naturally cools down as it prepares for sleep, and maintaining a cool bedroom environment—typically between 60 to 67 degrees Fahrenheit—can help facilitate this process. Avoid heavy meals, caffeine, and alcohol close to bedtime, as these can disrupt your sleep by either making it harder to fall asleep or by fragmenting your sleep throughout the night.

For those who find it challenging to unwind at the end of the day, incorporating a wind-down routine can be particularly beneficial. This could involve light stretching, journaling, or listening to calming music. The goal is to signal to your body that it's time to transition from the stresses of the day to a state of rest.

Advanced Sleep Techniques

Once you have mastered the basics of sleep hygiene, you may want to explore more advanced sleep techniques to further enhance your rest and recovery. These techniques are not for everyone, but for those looking to push the boundaries of conventional sleep, they offer intriguing possibilities.

One such technique is polyphasic sleep, which involves breaking sleep into multiple shorter periods throughout the day, rather than sleeping in a single long stretch at night. The idea behind polyphasic sleep is to reduce the total amount of sleep time while still getting enough deep and REM sleep to function effectively. Some of the most famous polyphasic sleep schedules include the Everyman and Uberman schedules, which involve taking several naps throughout the day. While some people swear by these schedules, they require strict adherence and may not be sustainable for everyone.

Lucid dreaming is another advanced sleep technique that can be both a fascinating and beneficial practice. Lucid dreaming occurs when you become aware that you are dreaming while still in the dream state, allowing you to control the dream's narrative and environment. This technique not only offers the potential for creative exploration and problem-solving but can also be used to address issues like recurring nightmares or anxiety. Practicing lucid dreaming involves techniques such as reality testing, where you regularly check throughout the day whether you are awake or dreaming, and keeping a dream journal to increase awareness of your dreams.

For those looking to enhance their sleep with supplements, there are several options that can support better sleep quality. Melatonin is one of the most popular sleep supplements, as it helps regulate your sleep-wake cycle, especially when adjusting to a new time zone or dealing with insomnia. Other supplements, such as magnesium, can help relax the body and promote deeper sleep. Herbal remedies like valerian root, chamomile, and passionflower have also been used traditionally to support relaxation and improve sleep. However, it's important to approach supplements with caution, as they can interact with other medications and may not be suitable for everyone. Consulting with a healthcare professional before starting any new supplement regimen is always a good idea.

Tracking and Analyzing Sleep

To truly optimize your sleep, it's essential to track and analyze your sleep patterns over time. This allows you to identify trends, make informed adjustments, and measure the effectiveness of any changes you implement. Fortunately, with the advent of wearable technology and sleep tracking apps, monitoring your sleep has never been easier.

Wearable devices like fitness trackers and smartwatches can provide detailed data on your sleep stages, sleep duration, and overall sleep quality. These devices typically use a combination of motion sensors, heart rate monitoring, and sometimes even oxygen levels to estimate the time spent in each stage of sleep. Some advanced models can also detect disturbances like snoring or sleep apnea, giving you a more comprehensive picture of your sleep health.

In addition to wearables, there are various apps designed to help you track and improve your sleep. These apps can analyze your sleep patterns, provide insights, and offer recommendations based on the data they collect. Many apps also include features like smart alarms, which wake you up during the lightest stage of sleep to help you feel more refreshed, and guided meditations to help you fall asleep faster.

When analyzing your sleep data, look for patterns and correlations. For example, you might notice that you sleep better on nights when you exercise earlier in the day, or that your sleep quality improves when you avoid caffeine in the afternoon. Use this information to make targeted adjustments to your routine and continue tracking to see how these changes impact your sleep.

The goal of tracking your sleep is not to become obsessed with the numbers but to use the data as a tool for making informed decisions about your sleep habits. Remember that sleep quality is just as important as sleep quantity, so focus on achieving a balance of both. Over time, with consistent tracking and a willingness to experiment with different techniques, you'll be able to fine-tune your sleep for peak performance.

Conclusion

Optimizing sleep is one of the most powerful steps you can take to enhance your overall performance and well-being. By understanding the science of sleep, implementing practical sleep hacks, exploring advanced techniques, and tracking your progress, you can unlock the full benefits of restful, restorative sleep. Whether your goal is to boost cognitive function, improve physical performance, or simply feel more energized throughout the day, prioritizing sleep will set the foundation for success in all areas of your life.

Chapter 3: Nutrition and Diet for Enhanced Vitality

- **Nutritional Foundations**

- **Biohacking Diets**

- **Supplementation and Nutraceuticals**

- **Personalized Nutrition**

Nutrition and diet are central pillars of biohacking, significantly influencing your energy levels, mental clarity, and overall health. By understanding the fundamentals of nutrition and exploring advanced dietary strategies, you can optimize your body's performance and enhance your vitality. This chapter will delve into the essentials of nutritional foundations, explore popular biohacking diets, discuss the role of supplementation and nutraceuticals, and offer guidance on personalized nutrition approaches tailored to your specific needs.

Nutritional Foundations

To build a solid foundation for optimizing your health through diet, it's essential to grasp the role of macronutrients and micronutrients and the concept of balanced eating.

Macronutrients—carbohydrates, proteins, and fats—are the primary nutrients that provide energy and support various bodily functions. Carbohydrates are the body's main source of energy, fueling everything from intense workouts to mental activities. However, not all carbohydrates are created equal. Complex carbohydrates, such as those found in whole grains, vegetables, and legumes, provide sustained energy and are rich in fiber, which aids digestion and supports overall health. In contrast, simple carbohydrates, found in sugary snacks and processed foods, can lead to rapid spikes and drops in blood sugar levels, which can affect energy and mood.

Proteins are crucial for building and repairing tissues, producing enzymes and hormones, and supporting immune function. Sources of high-quality protein include lean meats, fish, eggs, and plant-based options like beans and lentils. Adequate protein intake is vital for muscle maintenance and repair, especially if you engage in regular physical activity or strength training.

Fats, while often misunderstood, are essential for maintaining cell membrane integrity, hormone production, and absorbing fat-soluble vitamins. Healthy fats, such as those found in avocados, nuts, seeds, and olive oil, provide energy and support brain function. Omega-3 fatty acids, present in fatty fish like salmon and in flaxseeds and walnuts, are particularly beneficial for reducing inflammation and supporting heart health.

Micronutrients, including vitamins and minerals, are required in smaller amounts but are equally important for maintaining health and preventing deficiencies. Vitamins such as A, C, D, E, and the B-complex vitamins play critical roles in processes ranging from immune function to energy production and skin health. Minerals like calcium, magnesium, and iron are essential for bone health, muscle function, and oxygen transport, respectively. A varied and balanced diet rich in fruits, vegetables, whole grains, and lean proteins typically provides the necessary micronutrients, but individual needs may vary based on age, activity level, and health status.

Balanced eating involves combining these macronutrients and micronutrients in proportions that support your individual health goals. The balance can be adjusted based on factors such as metabolic rate, activity level, and specific health objectives. Ensuring a variety of nutrient-dense foods in your diet helps meet your nutritional needs and maintain overall well-being.

Biohacking Diets

Several popular diets align with biohacking principles, offering structured approaches to nutrition that can enhance various aspects of health and performance. Here's an overview of some prominent biohacking-friendly diets:

The ketogenic (keto) diet focuses on high-fat, moderate-protein, and very low-carbohydrate intake. By significantly reducing carbohydrate consumption, the keto diet forces the body into a state of ketosis, where it burns fat for energy instead of glucose. This metabolic shift can lead to improved fat loss, increased energy levels, and better mental clarity. The keto diet may be particularly beneficial for individuals looking to manage weight, improve metabolic health, or enhance cognitive function. However, it requires careful planning to ensure adequate intake of essential nutrients and to prevent potential side effects such as nutrient deficiencies or digestive issues.

The paleo diet emphasizes eating whole, unprocessed foods that mimic the dietary patterns of our pre-agricultural ancestors. This diet includes lean meats, fish, fruits, vegetables, nuts, and seeds, while excluding grains, legumes, dairy products, and processed foods. The paleo approach is based on the idea that modern health issues are a result of deviations from the diet our bodies are genetically adapted to. Benefits of the paleo diet include improved digestion, better blood sugar control, and enhanced energy levels. As with any diet, individual results may vary, and it's important to ensure nutritional adequacy while adhering to the paleo principles.

Intermittent fasting (IF) involves cycling between periods of eating and fasting, with various protocols such as the 16/8 method (16 hours of fasting followed by an 8-hour eating window) or the 5:2 method (eating normally for five days and restricting calories for two days). IF can lead to improved metabolic health, weight loss, and increased longevity by promoting cellular repair processes, optimizing insulin sensitivity, and reducing inflammation. While intermittent fasting is flexible and can be tailored to individual preferences, it's important to approach it in a way that supports your overall nutritional needs and lifestyle.

Each of these diets offers unique benefits and may be effective in different ways depending on individual goals and health conditions. Exploring these options can provide valuable insights into how different dietary approaches affect your body and mind, helping you make informed decisions about the best strategies for your personal biohacking journey.

Supplementation and Nutraceuticals

In addition to dietary changes, supplements and nutraceuticals can play a significant role in supporting health and cognitive function. These products can help fill nutritional gaps, enhance specific bodily functions, and optimize overall well-being.

Some essential supplements include:

- **Multivitamins**: A high-quality multivitamin can provide a broad spectrum of vitamins and minerals that might be lacking in your diet, supporting overall health and filling potential nutritional gaps.

- **Omega-3 Fatty Acids**: Supplements containing EPA and DHA, commonly found in fish oil, are known for their anti-inflammatory properties and benefits for heart and brain health. Omega-3s can help improve mood, cognitive function, and cardiovascular health.

- **Vitamin D**: Often referred to as the "sunshine vitamin," vitamin D is crucial for bone health, immune function, and mood regulation. Many people, especially those living in regions with limited sunlight, may benefit from vitamin D supplementation.

- **Probiotics**: These beneficial bacteria support digestive health and can positively influence immune function, mood, and even skin health. Probiotic supplements can help maintain a healthy gut microbiome, which plays a key role in overall wellness.

- **Adaptogens**: Adaptogenic herbs like ashwagandha, rhodiola, and holy basil can help the body adapt to stress and promote resilience. These herbs support balanced cortisol levels, reduce fatigue, and enhance mental clarity.

- **Nootropics**: For cognitive enhancement, nootropics such as bacopa monnieri, ginkgo biloba, and alpha-GPC can support memory, focus, and overall cognitive function. Nootropics can be particularly useful for improving mental performance and supporting brain health.

While supplements can be beneficial, they should complement, not replace, a balanced diet. It's important to choose high-quality products and consult with a healthcare professional before starting any new supplement regimen, particularly if you have existing health conditions or are taking other medications.

Personalized Nutrition

Personalized nutrition is the practice of tailoring dietary approaches to your unique needs, preferences, and goals. This approach goes beyond general dietary guidelines and takes into account individual factors such as genetics, metabolic health, activity level, and specific health objectives.

One effective way to personalize your nutrition is through biofeedback and testing. Biofeedback involves monitoring physiological responses to various dietary interventions and using that data to make informed adjustments. For example, tracking how your body responds to different macronutrient ratios or food types can help you identify which foods optimize your energy levels and performance.

Genetic testing is another tool that can provide insights into how your body processes nutrients and responds to different dietary patterns. Genetic testing can reveal predispositions to certain conditions, such as lactose intolerance or vitamin D deficiency, and guide your dietary choices accordingly. While genetic testing can provide valuable information, it should be used in conjunction with other methods and under the guidance of a healthcare professional.

Nutritional testing, such as blood tests for nutrient levels or food sensitivity testing, can also offer insights into your specific needs. These tests can help identify deficiencies or sensitivities that may be affecting your health and performance, allowing you to make targeted dietary adjustments.

Ultimately, personalized nutrition involves experimenting with different dietary approaches, monitoring your body's responses, and refining your strategy based on the data you collect. It's a dynamic process that requires ongoing attention and adjustment to achieve the best results.

Conclusion

Nutrition and diet are foundational elements of biohacking that significantly impact your vitality and performance. By understanding the basics of macronutrients and micronutrients, exploring biohacking-friendly diets, incorporating supplements and nutraceuticals, and personalizing your approach based on biofeedback and testing, you can optimize your diet to support your health and achieve your goals. The journey to enhanced vitality through nutrition is a continuous process of learning, experimenting, and adapting. Embrace this process with curiosity and an open mind, and you'll be well on your way to unlocking your full potential.

Chapter 4: Enhancing Cognitive Function

- **The Brain's Operating System**

- **Nootropics and Smart Drugs**

- **Mental Training Techniques**

- **Tracking Cognitive Performance**

Boosting cognitive function is essential for unlocking your brain's full potential, whether you're aiming to improve memory, enhance focus, or simply keep your mind sharp and agile. This chapter delves into understanding your brain's workings, exploring nootropics and smart drugs, practicing mental training techniques, and tracking your cognitive performance to help you achieve peak mental performance.

The Brain's Operating System

To enhance your cognitive function effectively, it's crucial to understand how your brain operates. Think of your brain as a complex, sophisticated computer with its own operating system. This "operating system" comprises billions of neurons that communicate with each other through electrical and chemical signals. These communications support various cognitive functions such as memory, focus, and decision-making.

The brain's ability to adapt and reorganize itself, known as neuroplasticity, is fundamental to cognitive enhancement. Neuroplasticity allows the brain to form new connections and pathways, improving its efficiency and functionality based on experiences and learning. By engaging in activities that challenge your brain, you can harness this plasticity to enhance cognitive abilities.

Understanding neurotransmitters is also key. Neurotransmitters are chemical messengers that transmit signals between neurons. Dopamine, for example, is associated with pleasure and motivation, while acetylcholine is crucial for learning and memory. By supporting the health and balance of these neurotransmitters, you can boost your cognitive performance.

Supporting brain health involves several lifestyle factors. A balanced diet rich in fruits, vegetables, whole grains, and lean proteins provides essential nutrients that support cognitive function. Omega-3 fatty acids, found in fish and flaxseeds, are particularly beneficial for brain health. Regular physical exercise increases blood flow to the brain, which is vital for maintaining cognitive function and promoting neurogenesis, the creation of new brain cells.

Sleep is another critical component. Quality sleep allows the brain to consolidate memories and perform essential repair work. During deep sleep, the brain removes waste products and strengthens neural connections, which is crucial for learning and memory. Aim for 7-9 hours of sleep per night, and establish a consistent sleep routine to support cognitive health.

Engaging in mentally stimulating activities can further support cognitive function. Learning new skills, solving puzzles, or playing strategic games challenges your brain and helps build cognitive reserves. Just as physical exercise strengthens muscles, mental exercise enhances cognitive resilience and flexibility.

Nootropics and Smart Drugs

Nootropics, or smart drugs, are substances that some people use to enhance cognitive function. These range from natural supplements to synthetic compounds. Nootropics are thought to improve various aspects of cognitive performance, including memory, focus, and mental clarity.

Natural nootropics include herbal supplements such as ginkgo biloba, Bacopa monnieri, and Rhodiola rosea. Ginkgo biloba is believed to improve blood flow to the brain, potentially enhancing memory and concentration. Bacopa monnieri is traditionally used to reduce anxiety and improve memory recall. Rhodiola rosea is known for its potential to reduce mental fatigue and enhance resilience to stress.

Synthetic nootropics, such as racetams and ampakines, are designed to enhance cognitive abilities by influencing neurotransmitter systems. Racetams, like piracetam and aniracetam, are thought to improve memory and learning by modulating acetylcholine receptors in the brain. Ampakines are another class of drugs that may enhance cognitive function by modulating glutamate receptors, which are involved in learning and memory processes.

While nootropics can offer cognitive benefits, they are not without risks. Synthetic nootropics, in particular, can have side effects and long-term health implications that are still being studied. Common side effects might include headaches, insomnia, or gastrointestinal discomfort. It's essential to use nootropics with caution, starting with low doses and monitoring your body's response. Consulting with a healthcare professional before adding nootropics to your routine is also advisable.

Combining nootropics with other cognitive-enhancing practices, such as a balanced diet, regular exercise, and sufficient sleep, can help maximize their benefits and reduce potential risks. Nootropics should be seen as a complementary tool rather than a replacement for healthy lifestyle practices.

Mental Training Techniques

Mental training techniques are another crucial aspect of enhancing cognitive function. Practices such as meditation and mindfulness can significantly impact brain health and cognitive performance.

Meditation involves focusing your mind and calming your thoughts to achieve a state of deep relaxation and heightened awareness. Regular meditation practice has been shown to increase gray matter density in the brain, particularly in areas related to attention, emotional regulation, and self-awareness. Even short daily sessions of meditation can lead to improved focus, reduced stress, and enhanced mental clarity.

Mindfulness is a form of meditation that emphasizes being fully present in the moment without judgment. Mindfulness practices can be integrated into daily activities, such as eating or walking, making them accessible and easy to incorporate into your routine. Research shows that mindfulness can improve attention, emotional regulation, and overall cognitive function by reducing stress and promoting a balanced mental state.

Cognitive training exercises, such as memory games, puzzles, and brain-training apps, are designed to challenge and improve specific cognitive skills. These activities can enhance memory, problem-solving abilities, and processing speed. It's important to choose exercises that are engaging and appropriately challenging to keep your brain stimulated and avoid boredom.

Physical exercise also plays a vital role in cognitive enhancement. Aerobic exercises like running, cycling, or swimming increase blood flow to the brain and support the growth of new brain cells. Regular physical activity has been linked to improved cognitive function, reduced risk of cognitive decline, and enhanced mood.

Combining physical exercise with mental training techniques creates a powerful approach to maintaining and improving cognitive function. The synergy between physical and mental activities supports overall brain health and contributes to optimal cognitive performance.

Tracking Cognitive Performance

To effectively enhance cognitive function, it's essential to track your progress and evaluate the impact of your strategies. Several tools and methods can help you measure different aspects of cognitive performance.

Cognitive assessment apps and online tests offer a way to gauge your memory, attention, and problem-solving skills. These tests can provide baseline data and track changes over time, helping you see how well your cognitive-enhancing strategies are working. Regular assessments can also help identify areas where you may need additional focus or adjustment.

Wearable devices and neurofeedback technology can provide real-time data on brain activity and cognitive performance. Neurofeedback uses sensors to measure brainwaves and offers feedback to help you regulate brain activity. This technique can be used to train specific cognitive functions, such as improving focus or managing stress. While neurofeedback can be effective, it's essential to approach it with realistic expectations and integrate it with other cognitive-enhancing practices.

Journaling is another useful tool for tracking cognitive performance. Keeping a daily log of your mental activities, mood, and any cognitive enhancement practices you're using can help you identify patterns and make adjustments. Reflecting on your experiences and noting any changes in cognitive function can provide valuable insights and help you fine-tune your strategies.

By using a combination of these tracking methods, you can gain a comprehensive understanding of your cognitive function and make informed decisions about your enhancement strategies. This data-driven approach allows you to optimize your cognitive performance and achieve your mental goals.

Conclusion

Enhancing cognitive function involves a multifaceted approach that includes understanding your brain's workings, using nootropics responsibly, practicing mental training techniques, and tracking your progress. By integrating these strategies into your routine, you can boost memory, improve focus, and achieve overall cognitive excellence. Embrace these techniques with curiosity and an open mind, and you'll be well on your way to unlocking your brain's full potential. Whether you're aiming to enhance your performance at work, improve your daily functioning, or simply keep your mind sharp, these strategies can help you achieve your cognitive goals and maintain a high level of mental well-being.

Chapter 5: Physical Fitness and Strength Optimization

- **The Science of Strength and Conditioning**

- **Biohacking Fitness Regimens**

- **Tech-Enhanced Fitness**

- **Recovery and Regeneration**

Maximizing physical fitness and strength isn't just about hitting the gym; it's about understanding how exercise impacts your entire body and mind. This chapter explores the science of strength and conditioning, provides strategies for optimizing your fitness routine, introduces technology to enhance your performance, and discusses effective recovery techniques. By diving deep into these areas, you'll learn how to enhance your overall well-being and mental clarity through a balanced approach to fitness.

The Science of Strength and Conditioning

At its core, strength and conditioning involve enhancing physical performance and overall health through exercise. To get the most out of your workouts, it's essential to understand how different types of exercise affect your body.

Strength training, which includes activities like lifting weights or doing bodyweight exercises, is crucial for building muscle and improving strength. When you engage in strength training, you cause small tears in your muscle fibers. This process, called muscle hypertrophy, triggers repair mechanisms in your body that make your muscles stronger and more resilient. Over time, consistent strength training leads to increased muscle mass, enhanced strength, and improved physical performance.

Cardiovascular exercise, such as running, cycling, or swimming, works on a different set of physiological systems. Cardiovascular workouts improve the efficiency of your heart and lungs, boost circulation, and increase endurance. Engaging in regular cardio exercises helps regulate blood pressure, reduce the risk of chronic diseases like heart disease and diabetes, and improve overall cardiovascular health. Additionally, cardio exercises have cognitive benefits; they increase blood flow to the brain, which can enhance mental clarity and cognitive function.

Both strength training and cardiovascular exercise offer significant mental health benefits. Exercise stimulates the release of endorphins, the brain's "feel-good" chemicals, which can elevate your mood and reduce stress levels. Regular physical activity has been linked to improved memory, better concentration, and even the mitigation of symptoms associated with anxiety and depression. Incorporating a mix of these exercises into your routine ensures a holistic approach to both physical and mental health.

Biohacking Fitness Regimens

Biohacking your fitness regimen means applying scientific principles and optimization techniques to enhance your exercise routine. One effective strategy is High-Intensity Interval Training (HIIT). HIIT involves alternating between short bursts of intense exercise and periods of rest or low-intensity activity. This approach has been shown to improve cardiovascular fitness, burn fat more efficiently, and build muscle strength in a shorter amount of time compared to traditional steady-state cardio. HIIT workouts can be highly effective and time-efficient, making them a popular choice for busy individuals.

Resistance training is another cornerstone of an optimized fitness routine. This type of training includes exercises such as weightlifting, bodyweight exercises, and resistance band workouts. Resistance training not only builds muscle strength but also enhances bone density and boosts metabolism. Compound movements, which work multiple muscle groups simultaneously, are particularly beneficial. Exercises like squats, deadlifts, and bench presses engage several muscle groups and provide a comprehensive workout.

In addition to these techniques, recovery is a crucial aspect of any effective fitness regimen. Recovery allows your body to repair and adapt to the stresses placed on it during exercise. Adequate recovery helps prevent overtraining, reduces the risk of injury, and supports long-term progress. Incorporate rest days into your weekly schedule, and utilize techniques such as stretching, foam rolling, and massage to aid in muscle recovery and flexibility.

Periodizing your training can further optimize your results. Periodization involves varying the intensity, volume, and type of exercise over time to prevent plateaus and keep workouts engaging. For example, you might focus on strength training for a few weeks, followed by a period of HIIT, and then switch to endurance training. This approach helps continually challenge your body and avoid adaptation, leading to better overall progress.

Tech-Enhanced Fitness

Technology has revolutionized the way we approach fitness, offering tools and resources to track, analyze, and enhance physical performance. Wearable fitness trackers are one such tool that provides valuable insights into various aspects of your health and exercise. Devices like smartwatches and fitness bands can monitor metrics such as heart rate, steps taken, calories burned, and sleep quality. By analyzing this data, you can tailor your workouts, adjust your activity levels, and track your progress more effectively.

Fitness apps also play a significant role in optimizing your fitness routine. Many apps offer guided workouts, track exercise performance, and provide nutritional advice. Some apps integrate with wearable devices to give a comprehensive view of your health and fitness data. These apps can help you set goals, monitor progress, and stay motivated by offering personalized feedback and recommendations.

Virtual fitness platforms have become increasingly popular, providing a wide range of workout options from the comfort of your home. These platforms offer various classes, from yoga and pilates to high-intensity interval training (HIIT). The convenience of accessing workouts online, combined with interactive features and community support, makes it easier to maintain a consistent exercise routine. Virtual classes often include real-time feedback and guidance, helping you stay engaged and motivated.

Incorporating technology into your fitness regimen can enhance your training experience, provide valuable insights, and help you achieve your fitness goals more efficiently. By leveraging these tools, you can gain a better understanding of your performance and make data-driven decisions to optimize your workouts.

Recovery and Regeneration

Effective recovery is essential for maximizing the benefits of your fitness regimen and supporting long-term progress. Recovery techniques help your body repair and adapt to the stresses of exercise, preventing injuries and enhancing performance.

Sleep is one of the most critical aspects of recovery. During sleep, your body undergoes essential repair processes, including muscle recovery and hormone regulation. Aim for 7-9 hours of quality sleep each night to support optimal recovery and overall health. Establish a consistent sleep routine, create a relaxing bedtime environment, and avoid stimulants such as caffeine close to bedtime to improve sleep quality.

Nutrition also plays a crucial role in recovery. A balanced diet with adequate protein, carbohydrates, and healthy fats supports muscle repair and replenishes energy stores. After a workout, consume a meal or snack rich in protein and carbohydrates within 30-60 minutes to enhance muscle recovery and replenish glycogen levels. Staying hydrated is equally important; drinking plenty of water helps maintain fluid balance and supports overall recovery.

Advanced recovery tools can further support your efforts. Cryotherapy, which involves exposing the body to cold temperatures, is used to reduce inflammation and accelerate recovery. This technique is popular among athletes for alleviating muscle soreness and speeding up recovery time. Other advanced recovery tools include compression therapy, which uses inflatable sleeves to enhance circulation and reduce muscle soreness, and infrared saunas, which aid in muscle relaxation and detoxification.

In addition to these techniques, incorporating practices such as stretching, foam rolling, and massage can improve flexibility, reduce muscle tension, and enhance overall recovery. Regular stretching and foam rolling help maintain muscle health and prevent injuries, while massage therapy can relieve muscle soreness and improve blood flow.

Conclusion

Physical fitness and strength optimization involve a multifaceted approach that includes understanding the science of exercise, implementing effective training strategies, leveraging technology, and prioritizing recovery. By combining strength training, cardiovascular exercise, and advanced recovery techniques, you can achieve improved physical health, enhance mental sharpness, and reach your fitness goals. Embrace these principles and practices to maximize your performance, prevent injuries, and enjoy the benefits of a well-rounded fitness regimen. Whether you're an experienced athlete or just beginning your fitness journey, these strategies can help you optimize your health and well-being, ensuring you perform at your best both physically and mentally.

Chapter 6: Hormone Balance and Longevity

- **Understanding Hormones**

- **Biohacking Hormonal Health**

- **Anti-Aging and Longevity**

- **Hormone Testing and Monitoring**

Hormones are powerful chemical messengers that regulate various aspects of your health, from metabolism and mood to growth and reproduction. Maintaining a healthy hormonal balance is crucial for overall well-being, longevity, and performance. This chapter will explore the role hormones play in your body, offer strategies for optimizing hormonal health, discuss advanced biohacks for extending lifespan, and guide you on how to effectively test and monitor hormone levels.

Understanding Hormones

Hormones act as messengers that travel through your bloodstream to regulate many bodily functions. They are produced by glands such as the thyroid, adrenal glands, and pituitary gland, and influence almost every system in your body. Key hormones include insulin, which regulates blood sugar levels; cortisol, which manages stress and metabolism; estrogen and testosterone, which are critical for reproductive health and muscle function; and thyroid hormones, which control metabolism and energy levels.

The balance of these hormones is vital for maintaining health and performance. For instance, cortisol, often called the stress hormone, can affect your sleep, energy levels, and immune response. Excessive cortisol, usually due to chronic stress, can lead to weight gain, disrupted sleep, and decreased cognitive function. Conversely, inadequate cortisol production can result in fatigue, low blood pressure, and weakened immune function.

Estrogen and testosterone, while known primarily for their roles in reproductive health, also influence muscle mass, bone density, and mood. As people age, hormone levels naturally fluctuate, leading to potential issues such as decreased muscle mass, slower metabolism, and altered mood. Proper hormonal balance can help mitigate these changes and support overall well-being.

Understanding the role of hormones in your body helps highlight why maintaining hormonal balance is essential. By addressing hormonal imbalances, you can improve energy levels, enhance performance, and support healthy aging.

Biohacking Hormonal Health

Biohacking hormonal health involves using lifestyle changes, diet, and supplements to maintain or restore optimal hormone levels. Here's how you can approach this:

1. Lifestyle Modifications: Lifestyle plays a significant role in hormonal balance. Regular exercise is a powerful tool for optimizing hormones. Physical activity helps regulate insulin sensitivity, balance cortisol levels, and enhance overall mood. Aim for a mix of aerobic exercises, strength training, and flexibility exercises to support hormonal health.

Stress management is another crucial factor. Chronic stress can lead to hormonal imbalances, including elevated cortisol levels. Incorporate stress-reducing practices such as meditation, deep breathing exercises, and mindfulness into your daily routine. Engaging in activities you enjoy and ensuring you have time to relax can also help manage stress effectively.

Sleep is vital for hormonal health. Quality sleep supports the regulation of hormones like cortisol and melatonin, which influence sleep patterns. Establish a consistent sleep schedule, create a relaxing bedtime routine, and ensure your sleep environment is conducive to restful sleep.

2. Dietary Adjustments: Diet plays a critical role in hormonal health. Consuming a balanced diet rich in whole foods, including fruits, vegetables, lean proteins, and healthy fats, supports hormone production and balance. Specific nutrients can also influence hormonal health. For example, omega-3 fatty acids, found in fish and flaxseeds, help reduce inflammation and support overall hormone function.

Avoiding excessive sugar and processed foods can also help maintain hormonal balance. High sugar intake can lead to insulin resistance, which can disrupt hormonal balance. Focus on whole, nutrient-dense foods to support healthy metabolism and hormone levels.

3. Supplements: Certain supplements can support hormonal balance and overall health. For instance, magnesium helps regulate cortisol levels and supports relaxation and sleep. Adaptogenic herbs, such as ashwagandha and Rhodiola rosea, can help manage stress and support balanced cortisol levels. Additionally, vitamins such as B6 and D play a role in hormone production and regulation.

Always consult with a healthcare professional before starting any new supplements, as individual needs can vary and interactions with other medications or conditions should be considered.

Anti-Aging and Longevity

Biohacking for longevity focuses on extending your lifespan while promoting health and vitality as you age. Several advanced biohacks can help you achieve these goals:

1. **Nutritional Strategies:** Caloric restriction and intermittent fasting are two strategies that have been linked to increased lifespan and improved health markers. Caloric restriction involves reducing calorie intake without malnutrition, which has been shown to improve metabolic health and increase longevity in various studies. Intermittent fasting, which cycles between eating and fasting periods, can also support metabolic health and promote longevity.

2. Exercise and Physical Activity: Regular physical activity is one of the most effective biohacks for extending lifespan and promoting healthy aging. Exercise improves cardiovascular health, supports muscle mass, enhances cognitive function, and helps manage weight. Incorporate a mix of aerobic exercises, strength training, and flexibility workouts into your routine to support overall health and longevity.

3. Advanced Therapies: Emerging therapies such as senolytics and NAD+ boosters are gaining attention for their potential to promote longevity. Senolytics are compounds that target and remove senescent cells, which are damaged cells that accumulate with age and contribute to aging-related diseases. NAD+ boosters, such as nicotinamide riboside (NR) or nicotinamide mononucleotide (NMN), aim to support cellular energy production and improve metabolic function.

4. Genetic and Epigenetic Interventions: Advances in genomics and epigenetics are opening new avenues for extending lifespan. Genetic testing can provide insights into your predisposition to certain health conditions and help tailor preventative strategies. Epigenetic interventions focus on modifying gene expression through lifestyle changes, such as diet and exercise, to support healthy aging and longevity.

Hormone Testing and Monitoring

Testing and monitoring hormone levels is essential for understanding and managing your hormonal health. Several methods can help you assess your hormone levels and track changes over time:

1. Blood Tests: Blood tests are commonly used to measure hormone levels, including thyroid hormones, sex hormones (estrogen, testosterone), and adrenal hormones (cortisol). These tests provide a snapshot of your hormonal status and can help identify imbalances or deficiencies. Regular testing can help track changes and assess the effectiveness of any interventions or treatments.

2. Saliva Tests: Saliva tests are used to measure levels of hormones such as cortisol and sex hormones. These tests can be particularly useful for assessing cortisol levels throughout the day, providing insights into your stress response and adrenal function.

3. Urine Tests: Urine tests can assess hormone metabolites and provide information about hormone metabolism and excretion. These tests can be used to evaluate hormone levels over a 24-hour period and offer insights into your overall hormonal balance.

4. Monitoring and Adjusting: Regular monitoring of hormone levels allows you to track progress and make informed adjustments to your lifestyle, diet, or supplementation. Work with a healthcare professional to interpret your test results and develop a personalized plan to address any imbalances or deficiencies.

Conclusion

Hormone balance is crucial for maintaining health, optimizing performance, and promoting longevity. By understanding the role of hormones, implementing biohacking strategies for hormonal health, exploring advanced techniques for extending lifespan, and effectively testing and monitoring hormone levels, you can enhance your well-being and support healthy aging. Embrace these approaches to maintain hormonal balance, improve your overall health, and achieve a vibrant and fulfilling life. Whether you're looking to optimize performance, manage stress, or extend your lifespan, these strategies provide a comprehensive framework for achieving your health and longevity goals.

Chapter 7: Environmental Optimization

- **The Impact of Your Environment**

- **Creating a Biohacked Environment**

- **EMF Exposure and Mitigation**

- **Biophilic Design**

Your environment profoundly impacts your health, productivity, and overall well-being. The spaces you live and work in can either enhance or hinder your daily performance and health. In this chapter, we'll delve into how your surroundings affect you, provide practical tips for optimizing your home and workspace, address concerns related to electromagnetic fields (EMFs), and explore biophilic design to create a more harmonious living and working environment.

The Impact of Your Environment

Your environment encompasses everything from the air you breathe and the lighting you experience to the ergonomics of your workspace. These factors can significantly influence your physical health, mental clarity, and overall well-being.

Lighting is a crucial aspect of your environment. Natural light exposure plays a significant role in regulating your circadian rhythm, which controls your sleep-wake cycle. Natural light helps synchronize your internal clock, leading to improved sleep quality, mood, and overall energy levels. Conversely, excessive exposure to artificial light, especially blue light from screens, can disrupt your circadian rhythm, leading to problems such as insomnia and reduced alertness.

Air quality is another important consideration. Poor indoor air quality can lead to a host of health issues, including respiratory problems, allergies, and diminished cognitive function. Common indoor pollutants include dust, mold, and volatile organic compounds (VOCs) from household products. Improving air quality can be achieved through measures such as using air purifiers with HEPA filters, ensuring proper ventilation, and incorporating indoor plants that naturally filter the air.

Ergonomics is the science of designing workspaces to fit human needs and capabilities. An ergonomically optimized workspace can prevent discomfort, enhance productivity, and reduce the risk of repetitive strain injuries. For example, an adjustable chair that supports proper posture, a desk at the right height, and a monitor positioned to reduce neck strain are essential for a comfortable and efficient workspace. Proper ergonomics can make a significant difference in your daily comfort and long-term health.

Creating a Biohacked Environment

Creating a biohacked environment involves making thoughtful adjustments to enhance your health, productivity, and comfort. Here are some practical strategies to consider:

Lighting Optimization: Start by maximizing natural light exposure. Position your workspace near windows to benefit from daylight, which can improve mood and productivity. During the day, open curtains or blinds to let in as much natural light as possible. In the evening, shift to warmer, dimmer lighting to avoid disrupting your circadian rhythm. Consider using dimmable lights or lamps with adjustable color temperatures to create a relaxing environment before bedtime.

To counteract the effects of artificial blue light, especially if you work late into the evening, consider using blue light filters on your screens or wearing blue light-blocking glasses. These measures can help reduce the impact on your sleep-wake cycle and improve your overall sleep quality.

Air Quality Improvement: Investing in a good air purifier can significantly enhance indoor air quality by removing pollutants, allergens, and particulate matter from the air. Look for purifiers with HEPA filters, which are effective at capturing small particles. Regularly clean and maintain your air purifier to ensure it functions optimally.

Ventilation is also key to maintaining good air quality. Whenever possible, open windows to allow fresh air to circulate, especially in areas where cooking or cleaning occurs. For homes in areas with poor outdoor air quality, consider using air exchange systems that bring in filtered outdoor air while keeping pollutants out.

Indoor plants can be a natural way to improve air quality. Plants like the snake plant, spider plant, and peace lily are known for their ability to filter indoor air pollutants. They also add a touch of nature to your space, creating a more pleasant and calming environment.

Ergonomics and Comfort: Ensuring that your workspace is ergonomically designed can greatly impact your comfort and productivity. Invest in a chair that provides good lumbar support and promotes proper posture. Your desk should be at a height that allows your arms to rest comfortably while typing, and your monitor should be positioned at eye level to reduce neck strain.

Consider incorporating standing desks or desk converters that allow you to alternate between sitting and standing. This can help reduce the risks associated with prolonged sitting and improve circulation. Ergonomic accessories, such as a keyboard tray or a mouse pad with wrist support, can further enhance your comfort and reduce strain.

Noise Management: Noise can be a significant distraction and stressor in any environment. If you find yourself in a noisy setting, noise-canceling headphones or earplugs can help maintain focus and reduce stress. Additionally, consider using soundproofing solutions, such as acoustic panels, to minimize external noise and create a quieter workspace. White noise machines can also be effective in masking disruptive sounds and creating a more serene environment.

EMF Exposure and Mitigation

Electromagnetic fields (EMFs) are generated by many modern electronic devices, including cell phones, computers, and Wi-Fi routers. While the research on long-term health effects of EMF exposure is ongoing, some studies suggest potential risks such as sleep disturbances, increased stress, and possible impacts on cellular health.

To manage and reduce EMF exposure, consider several strategies. One approach is to minimize the proximity of EMF-emitting devices to your body. For example, avoid carrying your cell phone directly against your body, and use speakerphone or wireless headsets to reduce direct contact during calls. Keeping devices like laptops and tablets away from your body when they are in use can also help reduce exposure.

Reducing reliance on Wi-Fi and opting for wired internet connections can further decrease your exposure to EMFs. If you use Wi-Fi regularly, consider turning off the router when it is not in use, especially at night. Additionally, creating EMF-free zones in your home, such as the bedroom, can contribute to a healthier environment for rest and relaxation.

There are also various EMF-reducing products available, such as shielding cases for phones and EMF-blocking clothing. Research these products carefully to ensure they are effective and suitable for your needs. Using these products in conjunction with other mitigation strategies can help manage your overall EMF exposure.

Biophilic Design

Biophilic design involves incorporating elements of nature into your living and working spaces to enhance well-being and productivity. The concept is based on the idea that humans have an innate connection to nature, and integrating natural elements into our environments can have various benefits, including reduced stress and improved cognitive function.

One way to implement biophilic design is by incorporating natural materials into your decor. Materials such as wood, stone, and natural fibers can create a calming and aesthetically pleasing environment. For example, wooden furniture or stone accents can bring a touch of nature indoors, contributing to a more harmonious space.

Indoor plants are another effective way to bring nature into your environment. Adding a variety of plants to your home or office can improve air quality and create a more inviting atmosphere. Plants like succulents, ferns, and herbs are not only easy to care for but also add greenery and a sense of tranquility to your space.

Maximizing natural light is also a key aspect of biophilic design. Use large windows, skylights, or light tubes to increase the amount of natural light in your spaces. This can help regulate your circadian rhythm, improve mood, and enhance overall well-being. Additionally, positioning your workspace or living area to offer views of outdoor greenery or natural landscapes can further enhance your connection with nature.

Conclusion

Optimizing your environment is essential for enhancing health, productivity, and overall well-being. By understanding the impact of lighting, air quality, ergonomics, and EMF exposure, you can make informed adjustments to create a more supportive and healthy environment. Incorporating biophilic design elements, such as natural materials and indoor plants, can further improve your living and working spaces, promoting a more harmonious and balanced lifestyle. Embracing these environmental optimization strategies will help you create a space that supports your physical health, mental clarity, and overall quality of life, leading to a more fulfilling and productive daily experience. Whether you're redesigning your home, setting up a new office, or simply looking to enhance your existing space, these insights offer valuable guidance for achieving a healthier and more optimized environment.

Chapter 8: Mastering Stress and Emotional Well-Being

- **The Physiology of Stress**

- **Stress-Reduction Techniques**

- **Cultivating Emotional Resilience**

- **Biohacking Happiness**

Stress and emotional well-being are central to achieving a balanced and fulfilling life. Understanding how stress affects the body and mind, and learning effective strategies to manage it, can profoundly impact your overall health and happiness. In this chapter, we'll explore the physiology of stress, practical techniques for reducing stress, ways to cultivate emotional resilience, and how to use biohacking to enhance happiness and emotional well-being.

The Physiology of Stress

Stress, though a natural and sometimes beneficial response, can have far-reaching effects on both the body and mind. When faced with a stressor, the body initiates a "fight-or-flight" response, releasing hormones like adrenaline and cortisol. These hormones prepare the body to respond to the perceived threat by increasing heart rate, elevating blood pressure, and redirecting energy to muscles. While this response is useful in acute situations, chronic stress can lead to negative health outcomes.

Prolonged stress can have several detrimental effects on your body. For instance, elevated cortisol levels over time can impair immune function, making you more susceptible to illness. It can also lead to weight gain, particularly around the abdomen, as high cortisol levels can stimulate appetite and increase fat storage. Additionally, chronic stress can contribute to cardiovascular problems, digestive issues, and mental health conditions such as anxiety and depression.

On a psychological level, ongoing stress can affect cognitive functions, such as memory and concentration. It can also lead to emotional exhaustion, irritability, and decreased overall life satisfaction. Understanding these effects is crucial for recognizing the importance of stress management and developing strategies to mitigate its impact.

Stress-Reduction Techniques

Effective stress management is essential for maintaining overall health and well-being. Several biohacking techniques can help reduce stress and improve your ability to cope with life's challenges.

Breathing Exercises: One of the simplest and most effective ways to manage stress is through controlled breathing techniques. Deep breathing exercises, such as diaphragmatic breathing, help activate the parasympathetic nervous system, which counters the stress response and promotes relaxation. Techniques like box breathing—inhale for four seconds, hold for four seconds, exhale for four seconds, and hold for another four seconds—can quickly calm your mind and reduce stress levels.

Cold Exposure: Cold exposure, such as taking cold showers or immersing yourself in cold water, is another biohack that can help manage stress. Cold exposure triggers the release of endorphins, which are natural mood enhancers. It also stimulates the vagus nerve, which can help regulate the body's stress response and promote a sense of calm. Gradually incorporating cold exposure into your routine can help improve resilience to stress and enhance overall well-being.

Adaptogens: Adaptogens are natural substances that help the body adapt to stress and maintain balance. Herbs such as ashwagandha, rhodiola, and holy basil have been shown to support the body's stress response and reduce the impact of stress on mental and physical health. Incorporating adaptogenic herbs into your daily routine can enhance your ability to handle stress and improve overall emotional resilience.

Exercise: Regular physical activity is another effective stress-reduction technique. Exercise increases the production of endorphins, which are known as "feel-good" hormones. It also helps reduce cortisol levels and promotes better sleep, both of which are important for managing stress. Engaging in activities you enjoy, whether it's running, yoga, or dancing, can provide a natural outlet for stress and improve your mood.

Cultivating Emotional Resilience

Emotional resilience is the ability to bounce back from adversity and maintain a positive outlook despite life's challenges. Developing resilience can help you navigate stress more effectively and improve your overall emotional well-being.

Mindfulness: Mindfulness practices, such as meditation and mindfulness-based stress reduction (MBSR), can significantly enhance emotional resilience. Mindfulness involves paying attention to the present moment without judgment, which can help you become more aware of your thoughts and emotions. Regular mindfulness practice can reduce stress, improve emotional regulation, and increase your overall sense of well-being.

Positive Psychology: Positive psychology focuses on cultivating positive emotions and strengths to enhance overall happiness and life satisfaction. Practices such as gratitude journaling, where you regularly write down things you are grateful for, can shift your focus from stressors to positive aspects of your life. Engaging in activities that promote joy, such as hobbies or spending time with loved ones, can also contribute to greater emotional resilience.

Building Support Networks: Having a strong support network of friends, family, or colleagues can provide emotional support and practical help during stressful times. Building and maintaining positive relationships can offer a sense of connection and reduce feelings of isolation.

It's important to nurture these relationships and seek support when needed.

Setting Boundaries: Learning to set healthy boundaries is crucial for maintaining emotional well-being. It involves recognizing your limits and being assertive about your needs and priorities. Setting boundaries in personal and professional life can help prevent burnout, reduce stress, and ensure that you have time for self-care and relaxation.

Biohacking Happiness

Biohacking happiness involves using scientific insights and techniques to enhance your emotional well-being. The science of happiness explores how various factors contribute to a positive and fulfilling life, and biohacking provides practical methods to improve your happiness levels.

Gratitude Practices: Research has shown that practicing gratitude can enhance overall happiness and well-being. Simple techniques, such as keeping a gratitude journal or expressing appreciation to others, can shift your focus from negative experiences to positive aspects of your life. Gratitude practices have been linked to improved mood, better relationships, and greater life satisfaction.

Positive Affirmations: Positive affirmations involve repeating positive statements about yourself and your life to foster a more optimistic mindset. By consistently affirming positive beliefs, you can reframe negative thought patterns and boost your self-esteem. Incorporating positive affirmations into your daily routine can enhance your overall sense of happiness and well-being.

Purpose and Meaning: Finding purpose and meaning in life can contribute significantly to happiness. Engaging in activities that align with your values and passions can provide a sense of fulfillment and satisfaction. Whether it's through work, hobbies, or volunteering, pursuing goals that are meaningful to you can enhance your overall sense of happiness.

Social Connection: Building and maintaining strong social connections is essential for emotional well-being. Positive social interactions, whether with friends, family, or community groups, can provide support, increase feelings of belonging, and enhance overall happiness. Investing time in nurturing relationships and engaging in social activities can contribute to a more joyful and fulfilling life.

Conclusion

Mastering stress and enhancing emotional well-being are essential for leading a balanced and fulfilling life. By understanding the impact of stress on your body and mind, implementing effective stress-reduction techniques, cultivating emotional resilience, and using biohacking strategies to boost happiness, you can improve your overall health and well-being. Embrace these practices and techniques to create a more resilient, joyful, and balanced life. Whether through mindfulness, positive psychology, or practical biohacking methods, taking proactive steps to manage stress and enhance emotional well-being can lead to a more satisfying and enriched experience.

Chapter 9: Tracking Progress and Analyzing Data

- **The Power of Data in Biohacking**

- **Tools and Technologies for Self-Tracking**

- **Interpreting Results and Making Adjustments**

- **Building a Personal Dashboard**

In the realm of biohacking, data isn't just numbers and graphs; it's the compass that guides your journey toward optimizing your body and mind. Tracking progress and analyzing data are crucial steps in refining your biohacking strategies, allowing you to understand what's working, what needs adjustment, and how to maximize your health and performance outcomes. This chapter delves into the significance of self-tracking, explores the tools and technologies available for monitoring various aspects of health and performance, offers guidance on interpreting results, and provides insights into creating a personalized system for tracking and visualizing your biohacking progress.

The Power of Data in Biohacking

The foundation of effective biohacking lies in the ability to monitor and measure your progress. Data offers a clear picture of how different interventions impact your health and performance. By systematically collecting and analyzing data, you can gain insights into your body's responses to various biohacking practices, such as dietary changes, exercise routines, or sleep optimization techniques.

Self-tracking allows you to set benchmarks and evaluate the effectiveness of your strategies. For instance, if you're experimenting with a new diet, tracking changes in energy levels, sleep quality, or weight can provide valuable feedback on how well the diet is working. This data-driven approach helps in making informed decisions and adjustments based on objective evidence rather than subjective feelings alone.

Furthermore, data helps in identifying patterns and trends over time. It can reveal how your body responds to different stressors, activities, or lifestyle changes, allowing you to fine-tune your biohacking practices for better results. Without data, you may rely on trial and error, which can be time-consuming and less effective. By leveraging data, you can streamline your approach, minimize guesswork, and accelerate your journey toward optimized health and performance.

Tools and Technologies for Self-Tracking

The advent of technology has revolutionized the way we track our health and performance. A wide array of devices and applications is now available to help you monitor various aspects of your well-being. These tools range from wearable devices that track physical activity to apps that monitor sleep patterns or dietary intake.

Wearable fitness trackers are among the most popular tools for self-tracking. These devices, often worn on the wrist, provide real-time data on metrics such as heart rate, step count, calories burned, and even sleep quality. Brands like Fitbit, Garmin, and Apple Watch offer sophisticated features that allow you to monitor your daily activity levels and assess your progress over time. Many of these devices also integrate with other health apps, providing a comprehensive view of your health metrics in one place.

Smart scales are another useful tool for tracking health data. These scales not only measure weight but also provide insights into body composition, such as body fat percentage, muscle mass, and water weight. This information can be particularly valuable for those focused on body composition changes or tracking the effects of a new exercise regimen.

Sleep trackers, whether incorporated into wearables or standalone devices, provide detailed insights into sleep patterns and quality. They can monitor variables like sleep duration, sleep stages, and interruptions, helping you understand how well you're resting and whether adjustments are needed to improve sleep quality.

Nutrition and diet tracking apps are also essential for those looking to optimize their dietary intake. Apps like MyFitnessPal or Cronometer allow you to log your meals, track nutrient intake, and assess the balance of macronutrients and micronutrients. This data can help you make informed dietary choices and understand how your nutrition impacts your overall health and performance.

Interpreting Results and Making Adjustments

Collecting data is just the beginning; interpreting it and making informed adjustments are where the real work begins. Once you have gathered data from various tools and devices, the next step is to analyze it to understand what it reveals about your health and performance.

Start by looking for patterns and correlations in your data. For example, if you notice that your energy levels are consistently lower on days when you have poor sleep quality, this indicates a direct relationship between sleep and energy. Similarly, if dietary changes lead to improvements in mood or cognitive function, this can guide future dietary decisions.

It's also important to consider the context when interpreting your data. Short-term fluctuations are normal, and a single data point may not provide a complete picture. Look at trends over time to get a clearer understanding of how your biohacking practices are impacting your health. For instance, if you're tracking physical fitness, assess your progress over several weeks or months rather than focusing on daily variations.

Based on your data analysis, make adjustments to your biohacking strategies as needed. If a particular approach is yielding positive results, consider enhancing or maintaining that practice. Conversely, if certain interventions are not producing the desired effects, it may be time to re-evaluate and try alternative methods. The goal is to continuously refine your strategies to achieve the best possible outcomes.

Building a Personal Dashboard

Creating a personalized system for tracking and visualizing your biohacking progress can greatly enhance your ability to manage and optimize your health and performance. A personal dashboard serves as a central hub where you can compile data from various sources and visualize trends and progress in a meaningful way.

Begin by selecting the metrics that are most relevant to your goals. These might include physical activity, sleep quality, nutrition, stress levels, or cognitive performance. Choose tools and devices that can provide data on these metrics and ensure they are compatible with your preferred dashboard platform.

Many digital platforms and apps offer customizable dashboards where you can integrate data from different sources. Tools like Google Sheets, Microsoft Excel, or specialized health management apps allow you to create charts, graphs, and visualizations that reflect your progress. By setting up a personalized dashboard, you can easily track changes, monitor trends, and evaluate the impact of various biohacking practices.

Regularly review and update your dashboard to ensure it reflects your current goals and priorities. Incorporate new data as it becomes available and adjust your visualizations to highlight areas of focus. A well-organized dashboard can help you stay motivated and provide a clear overview of your progress, making it easier to identify successes and areas for improvement.

Conclusion

Tracking progress and analyzing data are fundamental components of effective biohacking. By leveraging self-tracking tools and technologies, you gain valuable insights into how different interventions impact your health and performance. Interpreting this data enables you to make informed adjustments, optimizing your biohacking strategies for better results. Creating a personalized dashboard to visualize and manage your progress provides a comprehensive view of your journey, helping you stay on track and motivated. Embrace the power of data as you continue to refine and enhance your biohacking practices, paving the way for a healthier, more optimized life.

Chapter 10: The Future of Biohacking

- **Emerging Technologies and Trends**

- **Ethical Considerations for the Future**

- **The Global Biohacking Community**

- **Becoming a Biohacker for Life**

Biohacking has evolved from a niche interest into a burgeoning field, blending technology, science, and personal wellness into a dynamic and rapidly advancing domain. As we look to the future, several emerging technologies and trends are poised to transform the landscape of biohacking. This chapter delves into these cutting-edge advancements, discusses the ethical considerations they bring, introduces the vibrant global biohacking community, and provides guidance on how to embrace biohacking as a lifelong journey of learning and adaptation.

Bryan Sherrell

Emerging Technologies and Trends

One of the most exciting frontiers in biohacking is the development of advanced technologies that push the boundaries of what's possible in optimizing human health and performance. CRISPR and gene editing represent significant breakthroughs in this area. CRISPR-Cas9, a revolutionary tool for genetic modification, allows scientists to edit genes with unprecedented precision. This technology has the potential to address genetic disorders, enhance physical and cognitive traits, and even extend human lifespan. As CRISPR continues to advance, it could open up new avenues for personalized biohacking interventions, enabling individuals to tailor their genetic makeup for optimal health and performance.

Another burgeoning trend is personalized medicine, which uses genetic and biometric data to tailor medical treatments to individual needs. By analyzing a person's genetic profile, healthcare providers can design customized treatment plans that are more effective and have fewer side effects. This personalized approach extends beyond medicine into lifestyle optimization, where data-driven recommendations can guide everything from diet and exercise to mental health strategies.

Wearable technology is also advancing rapidly, offering new ways to monitor and enhance our health. Innovations such as smart contact lenses, implantable sensors, and advanced biometric trackers provide real-time data on various physiological parameters. These technologies not only help in tracking health metrics but also in predicting and preventing potential issues before they become significant problems.

Artificial intelligence (AI) and machine learning are becoming integral to biohacking. AI algorithms can analyze vast amounts of health data to identify patterns, make predictions, and offer personalized recommendations. This technology enhances our ability to optimize health by providing insights that are often beyond human capacity to discern. From predicting disease risk to optimizing training regimens, AI is set to revolutionize the way we approach biohacking.

Ethical Considerations for the Future

As biohacking technology advances, it brings with it a host of ethical considerations that need to be carefully addressed. The potential for genetic editing, for instance, raises questions about the limits of human enhancement and the implications for future generations. While the ability to correct genetic disorders is a promising development, the possibility of using gene editing for nonmedical enhancements could lead to significant ethical dilemmas. Issues such as genetic privacy, consent, and the potential for creating genetic inequalities must be addressed as these technologies become more accessible.

The use of advanced biohacking technologies also brings concerns about data privacy. As we rely more on wearable devices and AI for health monitoring, the amount of personal data being collected is enormous. Ensuring that this data is stored securely, used ethically, and protected from unauthorized access is crucial. The biohacking community, along with regulators and technology developers, must work together to establish guidelines and standards that safeguard individual privacy while enabling the benefits of data-driven health optimization.

Another ethical concern involves the potential for misuse of biohacking technologies. As with any powerful tool, there is the risk that these technologies could be used unethically or irresponsibly. Ensuring that biohacking practices are conducted with integrity and respect for human rights is essential for fostering trust and ensuring that advancements benefit society as a whole.

The Global Biohacking Community

The global biohacking community is a vibrant and diverse network of individuals, researchers, and enthusiasts who are passionate about optimizing human health and performance. This community spans across continents and includes a range of activities, from informal meetups to international conferences.

Biohacking conferences, such as the Biohacker Summit and the Quantified Self Conference, bring together experts and enthusiasts to share knowledge, showcase innovations, and discuss the latest trends in the field. These events provide opportunities for networking, learning, and collaboration, fostering a sense of community and shared purpose among biohackers.

Online forums and social media platforms also play a significant role in connecting the biohacking community. Websites like Reddit and specialized biohacking forums provide spaces for individuals to discuss techniques, share experiences, and seek advice. Influential figures in the biohacking world, including researchers, practitioners, and thought leaders, contribute to these discussions, helping to advance the field and inspire others.

Joining the global biohacking community can offer valuable resources and support as you navigate your own biohacking journey. Engaging with like-minded individuals and staying informed about the latest developments can enhance your knowledge, provide new perspectives, and keep you motivated to pursue your health and performance goals.

Becoming a Biohacker for Life

Biohacking is not a destination but a lifelong journey of exploration and improvement. Embracing biohacking as a way of life involves a commitment to continuous learning, experimentation, and adaptation. The landscape of biohacking is constantly evolving, with new technologies, insights, and techniques emerging regularly.

To become a biohacker for life, cultivate a mindset of curiosity and openness. Stay informed about the latest advancements in the field, and be willing to experiment with new approaches to health and performance. Regularly assess your own progress, and be prepared to adjust your strategies based on new information and experiences.

Engage with the biohacking community to share your experiences, learn from others, and stay inspired. Whether through online forums, local meetups, or conferences, connecting with fellow biohackers can provide valuable support and insights.

Ultimately, the goal of biohacking is to enhance your overall quality of life, and this pursuit requires ongoing effort and adaptation. By staying informed, experimenting with new techniques, and embracing the principles of biohacking, you can continue to unlock your full potential and lead a healthier, more optimized life.

Conclusion

The future of biohacking is bright and full of promise, with emerging technologies and trends offering new possibilities for optimizing health and performance. As we navigate this evolving landscape, it's essential to consider the ethical implications and strive for responsible innovation. The global biohacking community provides a wealth of resources and support, fostering collaboration and advancement in the field. Embracing biohacking as a lifelong journey allows you to continually explore, learn, and adapt, ensuring that you remain at the forefront of personal optimization and well-being. As you look to the future, remember that biohacking is not just about enhancing your body and mind but about embracing a transformative approach to living your best life.

Conclusion: Embracing the Biohacker's Mindset

- **Reflecting on the Journey**

- **Staying Curious and Adaptable**

- **Your Path Forward**

- **Living Optimally**

As we conclude our exploration into the world of biohacking, it's essential to reflect on the journey we've undertaken and consider how to continue evolving within this fascinating field. Biohacking is not merely a set of techniques or strategies; it represents a mindset—a commitment to exploring and optimizing every aspect of our bodies and minds. By embracing this mindset, you can ensure that your biohacking journey is both transformational and enduring.

Reflecting on the Journey

Throughout this book, we've delved into the core principles of biohacking, from understanding the fundamentals to mastering advanced techniques. We've explored how optimizing sleep, nutrition, physical fitness, cognitive function, and emotional well-being can significantly enhance your overall health and performance. Each chapter has provided tools and insights designed to help you unlock your full potential and lead a more vibrant, balanced life.

One of the key lessons from our exploration is the importance of a holistic approach to biohacking. True optimization involves not just focusing on one aspect of health but integrating various elements into a cohesive strategy. By balancing physical health with mental and emotional well-being, you create a foundation for sustained growth and improvement.

Another vital insight is the value of data and self-tracking. The ability to monitor your progress and make data-driven adjustments is crucial for refining your biohacking practices. As you continue to collect and analyze data, you'll gain deeper insights into what works best for you, allowing you to fine-tune your strategies and achieve even greater results.

Finally, the ethical considerations and responsible use of biohacking technologies underscore the need for thoughtful and informed decision-making. As you explore new techniques and advancements, it's essential to remain aware of the potential impacts on your health and the broader implications for society.

Staying Curious and Adaptable

The journey of biohacking is far from static. To truly embrace the biohacker's mindset, it's crucial to remain curious and open-minded. The world of biohacking is continuously evolving, with new research, technologies, and techniques emerging regularly. By staying informed and curious, you can keep pace with these developments and incorporate innovative practices into your routine.

Adaptability is also a key component of successful biohacking. As you experiment with different strategies and gather data, you'll encounter both successes and challenges. Being adaptable means being willing to adjust your approach based on what you learn. It's about viewing each experiment as an opportunity for growth and remaining flexible in your pursuit of optimization.

Engage with new ideas, challenge your assumptions, and be open to exploring unconventional methods. This mindset will not only enhance your biohacking experience but also ensure that you continue to discover new ways to improve your health and performance.

Your Path Forward

As you look ahead, consider setting new goals and challenges for yourself. The journey of biohacking is ongoing, and there's always room for further exploration and improvement. Reflect on the areas where you've made progress and identify new aspects of your health and performance that you'd like to optimize.

Connecting with the broader biohacking community can provide valuable support and inspiration. Whether through online forums, local meetups, or conferences, engaging with fellow biohackers can offer fresh perspectives, new techniques, and a sense of camaraderie. Sharing your experiences and learning from others can enrich your biohacking journey and help you stay motivated.

Consider pursuing advanced biohacking techniques or exploring new technologies as they become available. As you continue to expand your knowledge and experiment with different strategies, you'll gain deeper insights into what works best for you and how to achieve your personal goals.

Living Optimally

Ultimately, biohacking is about more than just achieving specific health outcomes; it's about living your life to the fullest. By integrating biohacking practices into your daily routine, you're making a commitment to living the healthiest, happiest, and most fulfilled life possible. Embrace the principles of biohacking as a lifelong journey, and remember that the goal is to continually strive for improvement and balance.

Living optimally means taking a comprehensive approach to your well-being, addressing physical, mental, and emotional aspects of health. It involves setting goals, tracking progress, and making adjustments based on your evolving needs and experiences. It's about finding joy in the process of self-improvement and celebrating the milestones along the way.

As you continue on your biohacking journey, remember that the path to optimal living is unique to each individual. Stay true to your goals, remain open to new possibilities, and embrace the adventure of discovering what it means to live your best life. With a biohacker's mindset, you have the tools and knowledge to transform your health, enhance your performance, and achieve a sense of fulfillment that enriches every aspect of your life.

Glossary

- **Biohacking**: The practice of using science, technology, and self-experimentation to optimize physical and mental performance, health, and longevity.

- **Self-Experimentation**: The process of testing and modifying personal health practices or interventions to observe their effects on one's body and mind.

- **Optimization**: The act of making something as effective or functional as possible, often by refining and adjusting various factors.

- **Sleep Hygiene**: Practices and habits that are conducive to sleeping well on a regular basis, including maintaining a consistent sleep schedule and creating a restful environment.

- **Polyphasic Sleep**: A sleep pattern involving multiple short naps throughout the day rather than one long period of sleep at night.

- **Lucid Dreaming**: The ability to become aware of and control one's dreams while they are occurring.

- **Nootropics**: Substances or supplements that are believed to enhance cognitive function, such as memory, creativity, or motivation.

- **Smart Drugs**: Also known as nootropics, these are substances intended to improve cognitive performance.

- **Neurobiology**: The branch of biology that studies the nervous system and its impact on behavior and cognitive functions.

- **Gene Editing**: Techniques, such as CRISPR-Cas9, that allow for precise modifications of an organism's DNA to alter genetic traits.

- **Personalized Medicine**: Medical care tailored to the individual characteristics, needs, and preferences of a patient, often using genetic and biometric data.

- **Wearable Technology**: Electronic devices worn on the body that track health metrics such as activity levels, heart rate, or sleep patterns.

- **Biometrics**: Measurement and analysis of unique physical or behavioral characteristics, such as fingerprints, voice patterns, or biometric data, for identification or health monitoring.

- **Cryotherapy**: A treatment involving exposure to extremely cold temperatures to reduce inflammation and promote recovery.

- **Hormone Balance**: The state in which hormone levels are maintained within optimal ranges for health and well-being.

- **Adaptogens**: Natural substances believed to help the body adapt to stress and normalize physiological functions.

- **EMF (Electromagnetic Field)**: A field produced by electrically charged objects, which can affect biological systems and health.

- **Biophilic Design**: An approach to architecture and design that incorporates natural elements into indoor environments to enhance well-being and connection with nature.

- **CRISPR**: A genome-editing technology that allows for precise modification of DNA sequences in living organisms.

- **Gene Therapy**: A technique that involves altering genes within an individual's cells to treat or prevent disease.

- **Artificial Intelligence (AI)**: The simulation of human intelligence processes by machines, including learning, reasoning, and problem-solving.

- **Machine Learning**: A subset of AI that involves the use of algorithms and statistical models to enable computers to improve their performance on tasks through experience.

- **Quantified Self**: A movement that uses technology to collect data on various aspects of personal health and behavior to gain insights and improve quality of life.

- **Biofeedback**: A technique that uses electronic devices to monitor physiological functions and provide feedback to help individuals control these functions.

- **Nutraceuticals**: Products derived from food sources that provide health benefits beyond basic nutrition, such as supplements or functional foods.

- **Biomarkers**: Biological indicators, often measurable, used to assess health status or disease progression.

- **Personal Dashboard**: A customizable interface that consolidates and visualizes data from various sources to monitor and track progress towards personal goals.

- **Longevity**: The length of an individual's life, often studied in relation to factors that contribute to a longer and healthier lifespan.

- **Holistic Approach**: A perspective that considers the whole person, including physical, mental, and emotional aspects, rather than focusing on individual parts.

- **Biohacker**: An individual who engages in biohacking practices to optimize their health and performance through experimentation and technology.

Did You Enjoy This Book?

Dear Reader,

I hope this message finds you well. I wanted to take a moment to express my sincere gratitude for choosing to read *"The Biohacking Guide: Mastering the Art of Optimizing Your Body and Mind"*. It means the world to me that you've invested your time and trust in my work.

If you found *"The Biohacking Guide: Mastering the Art of Optimizing Your Body and Mind"* enjoyable and valuable, I would be immensely grateful if you could spare a few moments to leave a review on Amazon, Goodreads, etc. Your feedback not only helps other readers discover the book but also provides valuable insights for me as an author.

Whether it's a brief comment about what you liked most, how the book impacted you, or simply your overall impression, your review would make a significant difference. Your honest opinion is invaluable in helping me grow as a writer and in reaching more readers.

Bryan Sherrell

Thank you so much for your support and for being a part of this journey with me. Your reviews truly mean the world to me.

Warmest regards,

Bryan Sherrell

About the Author

Bryan Sherrell is a biohacking expert with over 16 years of experience in optimizing mind and body performance. His passion for self-improvement has led him to explore cutting-edge techniques in health, wellness, and cognitive enhancement. Known for his practical, science-based approach.

Dedicated to helping others unlock their full potential, Bryan's work focuses on sustainable and ethical methods for achieving peak performance. He continues to inspire and guide those seeking to take control of their health and live their best lives.